CAREERS IN
COSMETOLOGY

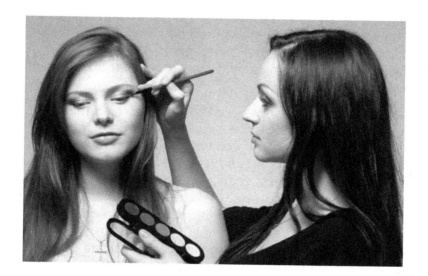

COSMETOLOGISTS ARE TRAINED TO MAINTAIN and care for hair, skin, and nails. Most are hair stylists, estheticians, nail technicians, or makeup artists. This is a very broad industry that offers numerous opportunities to specialize in very specific kinds of work. For example, a trained hair stylist might work only with wigs and hairpieces, or a makeup artist might work in live theater or for a local TV station. Most specializations are based on personal preference and experience, but some such as microdermabrasion or master coloring, require advanced training.

There are more than 600,000 of these professionals working in the US. That number is expected to rise faster than the average for the foreseeable future. The demand for licensed cosmetologists is greatest in hair salons and barber shops, nail salons, and day spas. There are also many jobs being created in resort hotels and department stores, on cruise ships and film and television sets, and backstage at fashion shows and magazine photo shoots. There are even traveling cosmetologists who bring their services to people in their own homes, assisted living facilities, hospitals, or small towns that do not have a salon.

There are many reasons people are attracted to this career. The main one is the easy entry requirements. College is not necessary. Cosmetologists do need to be licensed before working with clients, but that can be accomplished with less than a year of schooling and passing an exam. Most get their training in cosmetology schools, but some high schools offer cosmetology programs and there are online courses for those who need flexibility. There are also two-year associate degree programs offered by community colleges for those who want a more in-depth education.

The earnings potential is good for such a small investment in time. Most cosmetologists are paid hourly wages that add up to an overall average of about $30,000 a year. Since this is a service profession, tips are expected to boost one's income. It is also common to earn additional income from commissions by selling hair and skin products to clients. Motivated professionals have other opportunities to substantially increase earnings. Income can be much higher in big cities, especially in salons and spas catering to wealthy clients. In fact, a cosmetologist can double income with the right combination of location and employer. Cosmetology can be even more lucrative (in the six figure range) for motivated individuals who open their own salons, work with celebrities and actors, or market high end products by traveling to trade shows and conventions here and abroad.

If you are creative, good with people, and willing to keep learning more about your craft, this could be the right career choice for you. Cosmetology is a rock-solid profession that thrives even through economic downturns. Women and men always want to feel good about the way they look – almost more than anything else.

WHAT YOU CAN DO NOW

COSMETOLOGY SCHOOLS REQUIRE A high school diploma or GED. Unlike most colleges, there are no prerequisite courses. However, there are some types of classes that will be very helpful in preparing you for a successful career: communications, art, and science.

Communication is a vital part of cosmetology work. You will be interacting directly with clients all day long. To succeed in this career, you will need to understand what they want so you can give them what they are looking for. You need to know how to ask the right questions, listen closely to their answers, clarify what you think you heard, and make suggestions based on your knowledge and skills. You can learn much in English class, and speech and drama classes will provide you with useful techniques for interacting with strangers in a professional way.

Hone your innate creativity with art classes. Drawing, painting, and sculpture classes can teach you about color, textures, and aesthetics. Theater classes can provide you with opportunities to put classroom theories into action. You could work on costuming, set design, or even be the makeup artist for the cast.

If you are serious about this career, consider including biology, chemistry, and anatomy classes in your curriculum. It only makes sense to have knowledge of the human body when you are working with skin, hair, nails, feet, and hands. Estheticians providing facials, for example, need to know the location of facial muscles and all the nerves running to and from the head. Chemistry is involved, too, when mixing complicated colors or handling materials that could become caustic.

Visit college fairs. Along with four-year colleges and universities, you will find cosmetology schools. It is a good way to learn what the different schools have to offer. Be sure to ask representatives plenty of questions, such as what they teach, what advanced skills you could learn, and what their job placement record is.

Get experience. Experiment on your friends and volunteer to work on people who otherwise might not be able to obtain personal care services. This might include older people in nursing homes or assisted living centers or people who cannot afford such services but need to be presentable for job interviews. You can also get a part-time job in a salon. Sweeping floors and answering phones might not be glamorous, but it is the perfect way to learn what the day-to-day work is really like.

HISTORY OF THE CAREER

PERSONAL APPEARANCE HAS BEEN IMPORTANT to both women and men throughout history. Portraits and carvings of royalty and priests in ancient Mesopotamia showed that cosmetics were used long before the first century. Egyptian hieroglyphics indicate eyeshadow was used by the rich and elite – the "Cleopatra" look is still replicated today. Archeologists have uncovered ancient Egyptian makeup kits that included kohl and galena for eyeliner, crushed red ochre to redden lips, and red henna to stain fingernails and color hair.

Spas, manicures, and hairdressing originated in ancient Greece, and cosmetics were used for personal grooming on a daily basis. White lead and saffron was used to lighten the skin, kohl outlined eyes, and ground mineral cinnabar colored cheeks and lips.

The Romans embraced the Greek use of cosmetics and, in fact, were the first to commercialize them. A woman's class in society could be ascertained by the make-up she wore. Wealthy women had access to expensive cosmetics and lavish perfumes imported from China and Gaul, while poorer women could only afford cheaper products with life-shortening ingredients. Hair color also identified different classes: hair tinted red was high class, blond was middle class, and black was low class. At the famous Roman baths, clients were treated to saunas, massage, and various cosmetology services. More often than not, the masseuse, the nail dresser, and the hair stylist were slaves.

In ancient Asia, powdered lead was used for thousands of years to lighten the complexion of Chinese women. The Chinese also invented rouge for lips, but eventually phased it out in favor of a kind of black lipstick.

Cosmetics were only for the elite. The use of cosmetics by the lower classes was punishable by death. Neighboring Japan adopted the dark mouth fashion and took it one step further, using soot and ash to completely black out the teeth.

In the Middle Ages, makeup was forbidden, but that did not deter women from making their own from arsenic-laden white lead – a practice that often led to death. Fortunately, the rules changed during the Renaissance, and women no longer had to torture themselves to be fashionable. Plump bodies and fair skin, hair, and eyes were considered the ideal. Grooming was important for both women and men, and modernized cosmetology services were available even to middle class patrons.

Cosmetology trends and fashions evolved slowly throughout each era until the 20th century. At first, styles changed from decade to decade – a much faster pace than century to century, but by the end of World War II, styles were changing yearly and eventually only lasted a single season.

Modern Cosmetology in the US

Beauty salons are a relatively recent development. Prior to the 20th century, wealthy women had servants to take care of their hair and makeup. The majority of women tended to their own. Toward the end of the 19th century, cosmetology emerged as one of the few skilled occupations that provided women with the opportunity to become entrepreneurs. One such woman was Martha Matilda Harper. In 1888, she invented the first reclining shampoo chair and was the first to develop the idea of clients visiting a hair salon.

About 20 years later, Madam C. J. Walker established one of the most successful businesses in modern cosmetology. Born on a Southern cotton plantation, Madam Walker started out as a laundress, but became the first African-American woman millionaire. Her flagship product was a homemade treatment for hair loss, called the "Walker system." She went on to develop a line of cosmetic creams and hair products for black women, which she sold door to door. She marketed herself as a hairdresser and developed her own method of grooming based on her own products. As the products became more popular, she built up a sales force by training some of her customers to become "beauty culturists." Madam Walker eventually trained more than 20,000 women to provide her products and services across America and in several other countries.

One of the most enduring cosmetic lines, Max Factor, was introduced in 1909. It is named after a man who is credited for creating modern day makeup as we recognize it today. Max Factor's success came from simultaneously marketing makeup for movie actresses and everyday women. At about the same time, a teenaged entrepreneur, T. L. Williams, established Maybelline. The company's name was a mashup of Mabel, his sister's name, and Vaseline, which was the main ingredient in the company's first mascara. The 1920s was all about Chanel, red lips, and dark eyeliner. By the 1930s, two more cosmetic giants had emerged, L'Oréal and Revlon.

The professionalization of cosmetology began in the 1930s. Women, who were trained in small private shops, worked in crisp white uniforms. Their hair and makeup reflected the fashion of the time. Technology entered the picture, and cosmetologists operated electrical tools for the first time. Cosmetology services became increasingly popular during the 1940s. It was wartime and only professionals working in cosmetology shops had access to beauty products during this time. For that reason, cosmetologists were able to start supplementing their income by selling highly sought-after products to their clients on the side.

By the 1950s, the array of beauty products and tools was growing at breakneck speed. At first, there were hairspray and styling gels, blow dryers, electrolysis, electric curlers, and straightening irons. Then came hair extensions, permanent makeup, eyelash extensions, body contouring, and organic products.

Like all industries, scientific advances of the late 20th century moved cosmetology forward with techniques like microdermabrasion, scientific color matching, laser hair removal, and laser treatments for skin. Technology made it possible to provide personalized services, too. Today's high-end salons and spas are equipped with futuristic diagnostic tools like the microelectromechanical skin consultation system, and the various DNA tests used to customize skin care.

Technology and advanced training methods have also allowed cosmetology to become more specialized than ever before. For example, hair stylists can become master colorists, estheticians can offer medical-related services from doctors' offices, and nail technicians can specialize in artificial nail enhancement.

WHERE YOU WILL WORK

THERE ARE ROUGHLY 620,000 COSMETOLOGISTS at work in the US today. Most work in salons, spas, hotels, and resorts. A few work aboard cruise ships and a small percentage work in large department stores. Another small number of specialists work in funeral homes preparing the deceased for viewing.

There are also mobile cosmetology services. Traveling cosmetologists may be home-based, using an equipped van to visit clients in their homes, assisted care facilities, retirement communities, or hospital rooms.

About 40 percent of cosmetologists are self-employed. They may lease a booth or room from a salon or spa owner. Some will open their own shop after building a sustainable clientele.

Makeup artists may be self-employed, offering services to individual clients such as brides or celebrities. Some work in high-end salons and others are employed by performing arts companies or motion picture and television studios.

The work environment for cosmetologists is generally pleasant. High-end day spas and resorts, as well as salons in big cities can be very posh in order to attract the best clientele with money to spend on specialized services. At the low end there are tiny nail salons that may be sparsely furnished and smell strongly of chemicals.

Most cosmetologists work full time, but work schedules can be flexible. Part-time positions are common and arrangements are often made to work on an as-needed basis when there are bookings. Some salons and spas are open evenings and weekends to accommodate clients' schedules. Those who run their own shops can determine their own hours, but they often work long hours due to their business management responsibilities.

THE WORK YOU WILL DO

A COSMETOLOGIST IS SOMEONE WHO has been trained in the skillful cosmetic treatment of hair, skin, and/or nails. There is no single job description because the range of possible services is wide (and always expanding). Some do it all, but that is rare these days. Instead of performing general cosmetology services, these careerists typically specialize in one or more cosmetology services, such as hair styling, nail technology, skincare, or makeup.

Regardless of the type of services performed, there are basic tasks that every cosmetologist must do before and after seeing a client. At the beginning of the day, preparations start with reviewing the scheduled client list and requested services. Make sure everything needed to provide those services is at your workstation. It is important to have all the required products and tools ready, but it is doubly important for the safety and comfort of clients that the workstation be clean and tidy. Some clients will know exactly what they want, and others, not so much. Each appointment should begin by asking a lot of questions to learn what the client wants to accomplish. Once you are sure you understand what that is, you can begin service.

After services have been successfully rendered, propose a date for the next appointment. Most salons and their cosmetologists rely on retail sales for additional income. Do not wait for clients to ask – recommend they purchase the "special" professional products you just used to make them look fabulous. Before they leave, remind happy clients to tell their friends. Referrals are the number one way to build a thriving business. Be sure to keep records of hair color and skin care regimens for regular clients. Last, but certainly not least, thoroughly clean your work area and tools.

What any particular cosmetologist will do on a daily basis depends on what the chosen focus is.

Hair Styling

Hair stylists design, cut, shape, perm, color, and arrange hair according to the client's wishes and the latest fashion trends. They may also give advice on hair care and do scalp treatments. Some women go to a hair stylist on a regular basis. Others go when they need their hair to be especially nice for weddings, proms, or other special events.

Each individual is different and so is every client's hair, which can be fine, coarse, curly, straight, thick, long, or short. Choosing the most appropriate treatment and style also means taking into account the person's face shape, bone structure, skin tone, age, and lifestyle.

Hair styling sessions usually start with shampoo and conditioning. Hair stylists in most salons do this themselves. In large salons, this may be left to workers whose only task is to shampoo and condition hair before the stylist steps in and completes the service. Most people do not go to a salon just to get their hair shampooed, however, "blowout salons" have become popular in most major cities. These salons do not offer full services. Washing and blowing out hair is all they do. It is how many professional women maintain an attractive, polished appearance on a daily basis.

There are many options for hair stylists to specialize. Some specialize in certain types of hair, such as curly or long. Others specialize in extensions or straightening.

Some clean and style wigs and hairpieces. Most specializations are a matter of personal preference and experience. Colorists, however, receive advanced training and become board certified. Hair stylists can also be trained as barbers. They are trained to cut and trim men's hair, and may also provide beard trims, facial shaving, scalp treatments, and hairpiece fitting.

Nail Technology

Cosmetologists who focus on the art and care of fingernails and toenails, are known as nail techs. These professionals were previously known as manicurists, but as more and more services beyond simple manicures became available, that became too narrow a term.

In addition to manicures, nail techs may perform a variety of care and maintenance services on the hands including polish removal, cuticle treatments, polishing, nail trimming and shaping, nail art, and softening the skin of the hands. Similar treatments are applied to the feet. Some nail techs also provide hand and/or foot massage and aromatherapy. There are all kinds of artistic nail treatments, such as acrylic nails, gel nails, synthetic nails, and nail wraps.

Nail techs are trained to recognize diseases of the skin and nail, but they are not qualified to treat them. Instead, they would typically refer a client to a physician specializing in dermatology.

Skin Care

Cosmetologists who are trained to perform skin care treatments are known as estheticians. These are licensed professionals who are experts in maintaining and improving skin. Their most common service is the facial, which is the use of various cleansers, lotions, and oils to clean and soften the skin of the face. Other common services include hair removal, eyebrow shaping, massage, body treatments like wraps and hydrotherapy, chemical exfoliation, eyelash and eyebrow tinting, eyelash extensions, and aroma therapy.

Estheticians may receive additional training in certain machine-based treatments, such as laser hair removal, permanent makeup, electrolysis, microdermabrasion, electrotherapy treatments, LED, and ultrasound/ultrasonic. Any combination of these treatments might be used to perform non-surgical "face lifts."

Estheticians work mainly in day spas and resorts, but their advanced training also qualifies them to work in med spas and skin care clinics. They may provide consultations and treat a wide variety of skin issues, but only those that are cosmetic in nature, such as mild acne, hyperpigmentation, and aging skin. Skin disease and disorders must be referred to a dermatologist or other medical professional, even if the esthetician is working in a dermatologist's office.

Makeup

Estheticians are trained to apply makeup, but most makeup artists are not estheticians. Those who are estheticians usually limit their skin care treatments to facials and facial massage. Makeup artists are generally sought for special occasions, such as weddings, as well as special situations like male or senior makeup. They may also provide daily makeup services for celebrities in the public eye.

A makeup artist's tasks may include color pallet selection, eye and lip treatments, and application of facial foundation highlighted with blush or bronzer. They also provide instructions regarding the application of makeup, or recommend products and makeup colors to clients.

Some makeup artists specialize in theatrical and

performance makeup. This can be much more complicated because the play or film could be set in a different time period when styles were much different. They often have some homework to do to plan what will be needed and maybe even make some sketches or models. In many cases, they need to change the facial features of the actor altogether. To do this, they may also create special effects by using makeup to produce the illusion of aging or the presence of scars. In some cases, this requires the design of rubber or plastic prosthesis which they will attach to the actor before applying makeup.

Theatrical and performance makeup artists may apply makeup to actors themselves or instruct and supervise assistants in application and removal. They may also advise hairdressers to ensure that the hairstyles fit with the makeup.

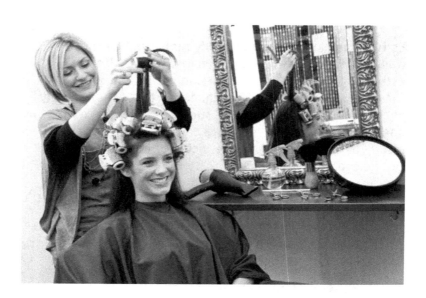

STORIES OF PEOPLE WORKING IN THE CAREER

I Am an Independent Esthetician

"I work out of a day spa when I have bookings, and the rest of the time, I provide services to people in their homes. My training in cosmetology school was specifically focused on becoming an esthetician. Since I gave my first facial 11 years ago, esthetics has become a well-respected profession. Doctors used to frown on the kind of work I do, but now many estheticians work from doctors' offices.

It wasn't long after I first started giving facials that I noticed how many people had serious concerns about their skin. My clients weren't just looking to be pampered with a spa day. They had persistent adult acne, rosacea, brown spots, wrinkles, and stubborn rashes that ruined their complexions. Many had been to dermatologists, but came away disappointed. Every night, I scoured the internet, trying to understand the various issues I was coming across. I needed to know what the possible causes were and how I could help. It took more learning than my formal training provided to dig out some of the answers, but my intense passion for learning paid off.

I have learned about all kinds of things that affect skin, like autoimmune conditions, aging, allergies, and sensitivity to things like gluten. Did you know that gluten is in almost every consumer cosmetic product? That's bad news for anyone who has celiac disease. I started to use only organic, gluten-free products and natural oils on my clients, and the results were amazing. I now have my own small skin care line that I make myself just for my clients.

This is a very emotionally rewarding profession. When I make people look good, I feel good. More and more people are interested in holistic health and that is what I can help them accomplish. The work is never boring. Every single client has different skin. Understanding their issues and treating the many aspects are satisfying, and sometimes even exciting – especially when they've tried so many other remedies."

I Work in a Neighborhood Salon

"I always wanted to be a hair stylist. I even had a doll-sized salon chair that fit my Barbie. So when my high school started offering a cosmetology program, I was all in. It was harder than I thought, with many extra hours of studying on top of my regular high school workload. My success depends on extensive knowledge in a multitude of areas. Everything I do involves a mix of art, science, and math. It took three years, but earning my license meant everything to me. That was five years ago, and I love my work now even more than I thought I would.

One of the best things about hairstyling is it's always advancing. There are new techniques, products, and tools introduced every day, and the styles are always changing. I need to be on top of what's going on in the industry, right down to who's doing what to their hair in Hollywood. It's a fun challenge for someone like me who's driven to be fashion forward.

This career offers a lot of freedom, both creative freedom and professional freedom. My clients come to me because they know I have an artistic bent that leans toward avant-garde. They trust my instincts and abilities, and allow me to try new cuts, use new techniques, and play with colors. Of course, whatever I do is designed to make my client attractive and happy, whether that's something sweet and elegant, or outrageously punk rock. Professionally, I have the freedom to choose my work environment, whether I want to specialize, and how much I want to work. I personally love being in a small, laid back salon where my neighbors come to have fun, swap stories, and leave looking fabulous. The relationships that blossom out of my work are irreplaceable. Even my best friend started out as a client."

PERSONAL QUALIFICATIONS

A GOOD COSMETOLOGIST CAN CUT AND COLOR HAIR, apply makeup, and perform other services according to what the client asks for. A *great* cosmetologist can create an entire new look that will help that person look attractive and fashionable. Both have skills, but the difference is the ability to visualize new ideas and incorporate changing styles and technologies in exciting ways that keep clients coming back. There are numerous other qualities that are also shared by successful cosmetologists.

Cosmetology is creative work. The best cosmetologists have an artistic flair that allows them to come up with new and different ways to apply their skills. They are able to determine what hairstyle and colors will complement each individual's bone structure, facial shape, skin tone, and hair texture. They find creative ways to help clients keep up with fashion trends while enhancing the personal attributes of each individual.

This is hands-on work that requires good manual dexterity. Like artists, cosmetologists must be able to perform intricate maneuvers and handle tools in positions that are sometimes awkward. Strength and stamina are also necessary. Working with cosmetology tools all day can be tiring for hands, arms, and shoulders. Mental discipline and physical stamina are needed to be able to be on your feet all day and still be cheerful with clients.

Like all service professionals, cosmetologists must foster customer service skills. Their success depends on building a repeat clientele. Successful cosmetologists have warm and sparkling personalities that make customers feel welcome and valued. They enjoy interacting with clients and go out of their way to remember names, details from previous chats, and personal preferences. A smile and a sense of humor also go a long way towards bringing clients back time and again.

Good listening skills are essential. The goal is to assess a client's needs and meet expectations. That starts with listening carefully to what clients say they want. It is common for clients to have trouble describing what they want. It can take patience to help them clarify what they mean so you can make sure they are happy with the results. Discretion is also important. Cosmetologists hear all kinds of personal stories that are not meant to be shared with anyone else.

Time management skills are needed to keep customers happy. No one likes waiting for service because the cosmetologist is "backed up." The cosmetologist should know how long a service will take to complete when scheduling appointments. Clients who receive timely care are more likely to return. Some services, such as hair coloring, require precise timing. It is not unusual for a cosmetologist to try and fit in a second client during the "downtime" of waiting for coloring or other chemicals to take effect. This kind of juggling can be disastrous if the cosmetologist is not able to manage the timing efficiently.

Good personal grooming habits are a basic necessity. This business is based on fashion and appearance. Think of yourself as a walking billboard for your services. A successful cosmetologist is always well-dressed, with a fashionable hairstyle and attractive makeup. It instills confidence in clients so they will trust your advice and want to return.

Tidiness is also a virtue. The work area, tools, and equipment should always be clean and sanitary. It is necessary for the health and safety of the clients, but also helps clients be comfortable.

ATTRACTIVE FEATURES

THE FIELD OF COSMETOLOGY HAS much to offer creative individuals with a passion for fashion and style. It has been consistently ranked high on the "Best Jobs" lists from US News & World Report in the service category. When asked why cosmetologists love the work they do, the first reason that comes up is the satisfaction that comes from helping people feel good about themselves. These professionals learn all the technical aspects of the job in school, but the sense of accomplishment and personal fulfillment does not come from simply graduating. It comes from sharing that knowledge with clients. Successful cosmetologists are skilled at bringing out the beauty in each individual client. The ultimate reward is the smile on the client's face. Here are some other reasons to choose this career path.

Fast Entry

Cosmetology has long been a popular choice for those wanting to get a career underway quickly after high school. It is not necessary to spend the time and money on a four-year college education. Most cosmetology training programs can be completed in as few as nine months. You can even get your training in high school or earn money while you train by working as an apprentice.

You Have Options

Cosmetology is a field that includes a wide range of services. In fact, there are no "generalists." Instead, cosmetologists can choose from a variety of services. Training for some, like hair styling, skin care, and nail technology, is offered in the regular cosmetology programs. There are also numerous specializations. These may require an additional six months of advanced training that will qualify you for professional certifications. Cosmetology skills are portable, and there is always an opportunity to change direction and pursue high-paying jobs that are typically reserved for certified specialists.

Job Security

There are plenty of jobs for cosmetologists and rapid job growth is in the forecast. Once in the field, cosmetologists do not need to be concerned about layoffs. The services they provide are all hands-on – there is no way to outsource the work overseas. Even recessions have little effect on employment. Cosmetology services are among the "affordable luxuries" that tend to perform well during economic downturns.

Flexibility

Cosmetologists are at work in every corner of the country, from the biggest cities to the tiniest towns. With the necessary license, it is possible to work wherever you choose. If life circumstances make it impossible to work full time, part-time work is a common option. There are several ways to work out a flexible schedule that can accommodate irregular hours.

Relationships

Cosmetologists interact with clients and colleagues all day every day. This creates an opportunity to build positive relationships with all kinds of people. Regular, long-term clients can easily turn into friends. It is also common to socialize with coworkers outside of work.

The Chance to Be Your Own Boss

About 44 percent of cosmetologists are self-employed. Some contract with existing businesses, renting work space in a salon, spa, or resort. Others are mobile, making house calls with virtually no overhead expense (except for their car). Still others open their own places of business. Being self-employed offers the freedom to make decisions about fees and work hours, but it does require good time and money management skills.

UNATTRACTIVE ASPECTS

THE COSMETOLOGY FIELD HAS MUCH TO OFFER, but it is not necessarily all good. Success in this career requires hard work and perseverance to get past some of the less-pleasing aspects. Before forging ahead with career plans, you should have a realistic view of what to expect. Here are a few possible downsides to consider:

Staying on top of the latest trends and styles can be fun, until it becomes work. Cosmetologists are expected to maintain an appearance that reflects their ability to provide fashion-forward services. This can become tiring, especially on those days when you just want to pull your hair back into a ponytail and wear something comfortable.

Cosmetology work can be physically tiring. The days can be long – sometimes 10 hours or more – especially when salons stay open late to accommodate clients with day jobs. Most of that time is spent standing and leaning over clients. This can be hard on the feet, legs, and lower back. Sore knees and shoulders are also common.

Depending on the type of services provided in the workplace, cosmetologists may be exposed to chemicals and dyes. Chemical solvents and dusts can be inhaled or ingested if hands are not carefully washed before eating. Even if the cosmetologist does not work directly with chemicals, there can be exposure due to the work of neighboring colleagues. The fumes from some chemicals in cosmetology products can carry throughout the establishment, irritating eyes and lungs and aggravating allergies.

It can be a joy to see the smile on the face of a happy client, but it simply is not possible to please everyone all the time. People are naturally vane and some have unreasonable expectations. Some can be unpleasant and others downright rude if they do not get exactly what they want. Cosmetologists have to be friendly and patient no matter what kind of person comes their way.

Most cosmetologists are not usually paid a salary, but instead earn an hourly wage. The median hourly wage is less than the national average for all other occupations. Sometimes it is only minimum wage, but there are also those who earn a decent amount. Like most service workers, cosmetologists depend on tips to supplement their income. Tips can be unpredictable though since not all customers follow the recommended guidelines of 10 to 15 percent for services. Tips also depend on the type of establishment, with high-end spas producing the most, and strip mall salons the lowest.

There are ways for cosmetologists to boost their income, but there are often obstacles. In many cases, they must pay rent on their workspaces. They need to build and maintain a steady clientele in order to cover the rent and make a good living. It can take some time to build a solid client base – two to three years is average. Moving to a higher-paying environment like a resort spa is a good idea, but there is stiff competition for those jobs. Commissions from selling products to clients can add income, but not everyone is cut out for sales. Cosmetologists are more often creative types and the pressure to sell can cause stress.

Cosmetologists do not generally receive the usual benefits other professionals expect. Those who are self-employed must provide their own health coverage and retirement savings. Even those who are not self-employed must work in order to make money. That means they are not paid if they are sick or on vacation.

EDUCATION AND TRAINING

ALL STATES REQUIRE COSMETOLOGISTS to complete an approved training program before starting work as a cosmetologist. In most cases, that means enrolling in an accredited cosmetology program. These programs are offered at independent Vo-Tech schools, community colleges, and some high schools. Only the high school programs are free, but typically the instruction is too basic to meet state requirements for licensing. An alternative is to take an online course, but the student would have to find a salon that would provide the opportunity to get the necessary experience.

Some states will accept an apprenticeship as substitution for cosmetology school. In this case, there will be a minimum number of hours of experience required and the cosmetologist will need to demonstrate satisfactory knowledge and skills by passing an exam. Additionally, some well-known salons operate their own specific training programs or institutes.

A full-time student in a cosmetology school can complete a typical cosmetology program in nine to 12 months. Typically, 1,000 to 1,500 hours of classroom instruction plus hands-on experience are required to complete any cosmetology program. Advanced specialist training takes about six months or an additional 600 hours of instruction. Community colleges offer two-year associate degree programs.

Training is short compared to many other careers, but that does not mean it is easy. The classes are condensed and the textbooks are huge and loaded with technical details. Many students do not pass the final exam on the first attempt. So take it seriously!

The curriculum is usually based on state licensing requirements, which can vary from state to state.

Actual coursework will depend on the student's career goals. For example, an aspiring esthetician would not receive the same training as a student preparing to become a hairstylist. The hairstyling program would cover principles of hair design, cutting and styling, color mixing and application techniques, scalp disorders and treatments, haircutting tools and devices, and chemical texture services. The esthetician would need to learn things like skin types, skin problems and solutions, facial techniques, product ingredients, makeup application, eyebrow shaping, and facial massage.

In addition to classroom instruction, cosmetology programs provide students with opportunities to practice what they have learned in class. Most cosmetology schools offer services at discounted rates to the public in order to provide experience for students.

Advanced Training

Students can choose to obtain advanced training in their specialized fields. In many cases, the training will make them eligible for additional certifications. For example, a hair stylist could become a certified colorist, or an esthetician could earn certifications in specialized procedures such as micropigmentation (facial tattooing like permanent eyeliner), chemical resurfacing, micro-dermabrasion, electrolysis, or certain massage services like reflexology.

Licensing and Certifications

All states require cosmetologists to be licensed. Precise requirements vary among states, but most require completing an accredited and state-approved program that provides adequate classroom instruction and a specified number of hours of practical experience. Upon graduation, the candidate will be eligible to take the state licensing exams. There are typically two parts, a written exam and a practical test. Written exams cover theories and procedures, sanitation rules, state laws, and basic knowledge of anatomy and chemistry. Practical tests involve performing requested services on a mannequin or live model. Some states also conduct an oral examination.

In many states, separate licenses are needed for each type of cosmetology, such as hair stylist, esthetician, or nail technologist. Others combine specialties under one unified license. It is also common for states to require licensing to practice in that state even when a cosmetologist has a license to work in another state.

There is usually a licensing fee, or even a fee just to take the test (whether you pass or not). Most states require you to renew your license regularly. That may mean filing appropriate paperwork and paying a renewal fee every couple of years.

In addition to state licensing, which is mandatory, there are also voluntary certifications. These are offered through professional associations and are usually meant to demonstrate superior expertise in a particular specialized service. Certifications give candidates a distinct advantage when applying for jobs. In some cases, employers will require certification for a particular position.

EARNINGS

MOST COSMETOLOGISTS ARE PAID AN HOURLY WAGE rather than an annual salary. Currently, the median hourly wage for all cosmetologists is roughly $12. The lowest 10 percent earn less than $9, and the highest 10 percent earn more than $24. On a yearly basis, the average is about $27,500. This amount does not necessarily include tips, which can boost earnings from 15 to 25 percent depending on the type of clientele.

How much any particular cosmetologist earns will vary by location, experience, and whether specialized services are offered. Geographical location can make a big difference in pay. The pay is generally higher in metropolitan areas than small towns or rural areas. For example, cosmetologists in Washington DC earn an average of $50,000 a year. That is nearly twice the national average. Other high-paying areas include Hawaii and California.

Earnings typically increase with experience. Newcomers might start out at minimum wage, but as they establish themselves and build a good reputation for quality service, earnings grow. Word of mouth recommendations are the lifeblood of this field. Employers rely on the reputation of their staff to draw more clients. They are therefore often willing to pay more to in-demand cosmetologists that clients specifically ask for by name. High quality work can elicit praise, and it also means bigger tips. In some affluent areas, it is not unusual for loyal clients to tip as much as the base price for service.

Obtaining advanced skills and offering specialized services are the surest way to earn top dollar in this field. There are several service types that can earn a cosmetologist more than $50,000 a year. For example, estheticians are among the top paid hands-on cosmetologists. The top 10 percent of these skincare specialists earn $60,000 or more per year.

The highest pay goes to makeup artists who work with performers, such as actors and singers. The training required to become certified in this area is not much different than any other cosmetology specialty, yet the potential earnings are much greater. The average annual wage is around $65,000 and motivated artists working in the right location can earn $100,000 or more per year. This is a specialization that is highly location dependent. There are a handful of cities where theatrical makeup is needed and pay reflects the demand for top professionals. New York City is one such location. Theatrical makeup artists there earn an average yearly salary of more than $90,000, and those at the top of their field are paid substantially more.

The Scheduling Effect

Many cosmetologists work part time on an "as needed" basis. This can be an attractive arrangement for those who need to work around school, other work schedules, or family obligations. Unless the cosmetologist has a sterling reputation and some loyal clients who are willing to be flexible, it can be hard to achieve higher earnings working only part time. On the flip side, some cosmetologists work evenings and weekends in order to accommodate clients' schedules. In some cases, these clients may be willing to pay a premium rate and tip more generously.

Cosmetologists cannot expect the usual benefits that other workers receive. Benefits are the exception rather than the rule for both regular staff and self-employed workers. They are responsible for providing their own health insurance and retirement plans.

OPPORTUNITIES

THE EMPLOYMENT OF COSMETOLOGISTS will continue its fast pace. Over the coming decade, the number of jobs is expected to increase more than 10 percent, which is faster than the average for all occupations. Most openings will arise from workers changing careers, retiring, or leaving the occupation for other reasons. There are plenty of candidates vying for jobs though, creating strong competition for positions. The toughest competition is at the higher paying spas and salons that can afford to be selective about who they hire.

Overall, job opportunities are expected to be good, but in some types of cosmetology they are better. Demand for specialty and advanced skin and hair treatments is on the rise – a trend that is expected to continue for the foreseeable future. Being a generalist with basic knowledge and skills might get you in the door, but you will not get very far without a sought-after specialization.

Skincare specialists, also known as estheticians, are in high demand. They typically work in high-end spas, performing treatments like facials, laser hair removal, waxing, and microdermabrasion. A highly skilled esthetician is able to build a solid clientele of repeat customers, which means more bookings and more tips. They may also receive a cut of the sales of premium products carried by the spa, bringing their total income to well over $50,000 a year. In short, estheticians can mean big business for the spas and vice versa.

Job growth will also be especially high for theatrical and production makeup artists. These specialists are looking at an increase of 15 percent over the coming decade.

Most of the new jobs will be in the motion picture and video industries. This also happens to be where makeup artists can earn the highest wages. High employment rates are also expected in personal care services (usually for celebrities), performing arts companies, and television broadcasting. These jobs tend to be clustered in New York, Illinois, California, Florida, Nevada, and Pennsylvania.

The future also looks bright for those who dream of opening their own spa or salon. This is a common step for experienced professionals who have built a lengthy client list, and have effectively outgrown their employer. There are several options available, including buying into a franchise business, buying out an existing business, or starting a new business from scratch. Assuming the prospective entrepreneur has a head for business management and a source of operating capital, ownership could mean a huge step up in earnings. Some spa or salon owners offset overhead by renting out styling chairs, facial rooms, or nail tech tables to independent professionals. Others might add a high-end line of products that clients pay top dollar for in hopes of replicating salon results at home.

GETTING STARTED

LAUNCHING YOUR CAREER IN COSMETOLOGY should not be difficult, but it can be if you are unprepared and have unrealistic expectations. For example, many cosmetology students assume their school is going to place them in a job upon graduation. That may be what the admissions representative say, but that is a general statement that may or may not mean you receive effective help in landing your first job. All prospective students should ask what the school's job placement rate is for graduates, before enrolling.

It is true that most schools offer some type of career placement services, but the services vary greatly. Most at least have job boards that post openings in the area near the school. School owners and instructors often have relationships with businesses in the community that are open to placing graduates if and when there are job openings available. That can be very helpful if you intend to work in the same area where your school is located.

Some schools have job placement coaches that can advise you on how to handle interviews, what your portfolio should look like, where the job fairs are, how to network effectively, and how to make yourself more attractive to employers. If this service is available at your school, start taking advantage of it well before graduation.

If you do not live near the school, you will need to put in some time and effort getting to know the potential employers in your community. Start this process while you are still in school. Introduce yourself to salon managers and spa owners and talk to them about your career goals. Let them know when you expect to have your license. Drop into the places where you would like to work from time to time so you become a familiar face. Developing relationships like this will give you a distinct advantage over unknown candidates when positions become available.

Make a habit of routinely checking online job boards. There you will find cosmetology positions posted on the general job sites like Indeed, CareerBuilder, and GlassDoor. There are also job sites devoted specifically to the various kinds of cosmetology. In either case, you can search for jobs, upload your résumé and/or portfolio, and apply directly.

A particularly effective online tool is LinkedIn. There you can build a profile that includes your résumé, portfolio, and references. Unlike most job boards where all you can do is upload a résumé, you can write about yourself and your career goals in any style and format you want. Once you have a LinkedIn profile, you can start making connections and joining groups that are relevant to your profession. Many employers and recruiters use LinkedIn to fill positions so do not be surprised if you start receiving offers seemingly out of the blue.

Use technology to your advantage by making your portfolio widely available. It is easy to create an online portfolio that showcases your best ideas. To impress employers, include both still images and a video of your work in action. Send a link to your online portfolio or attach an electronic version when contacting prospective employers. You can also use social media to build your visibility by posting short tutorials or demonstrations on YouTube, Instagram, or Pinterest.

Most students want to grab the first job that comes along after graduation, but you can beat out the competition for the very best jobs by making yourself more valuable. Take a little more time to get some advanced training from a well-known training company in men's hair shaping techniques, permanent makeup (facial tattoos), eyelash extensions, microdermabrasion, master color mixing, or even business building. The additional knowledge and skills gained through these classes will certainly set you apart from the typical newly graduated student. Plus, it demonstrates that you are serious about your career in cosmetology.

ASSOCIATIONS

■ **American Association of Cosmetology Schools**
http://www.beautyschools.org

■ **Professional Beauty Association**
https://probeauty.org

■ **National-Interstate Council of State Boards of Cosmetology**
https://nictesting.org

■ **The Day Spa Association**
http://www.dayspaassociation.com

■ **Professional Beauty Federation**
www.probeautyfederation.org

PERIODICALS

■ **American Salon**
http://www.americansalonmag.com

■ **Salon Today**
http://www.salontoday.com

■ **Modern Salon**
http://www.modernsalon.com

■ **NailPro**
http://www.nailpro.com

■ **Day Spa Magazine**
http://www.dayspamagazine.com

WEBSITES

■ **Cosmetology Schools**
http://www.cosmetology-schools.ws

■ **Beauty Schools Directory**
https://www.beautyschoolsdirectory.com

■ **Salon Channel**
http://www.salonchannel.com

CPSIA information can be obtained
at www.ICGtesting.com
Printed in the USA
LVHW082254290719
625809LV00015B/919/P

9 781722 428754